IF FOUND,
PLEASE RETURN TO:

NAME: Aidan & Brooke Hackett

ADDRESS:

PHONE NUMBER:

EMAIL:

LIVING
WELL
ONE LINE
A DAY

A FIVE-YEAR
REFLECTION
BOOK

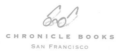

CHRONICLE BOOKS
SAN FRANCISCO

ISBN 978-1-4521-2548-0

Manufactured in China.

Designed by ANNE KENADY

10 9 8 7 6 5 4 3

Chronicle Books LLC
680 Second Street
San Francisco, California 94107

www.chroniclebooks.com

A comparative chronicle of your daily awakenings over the course of five years.

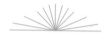

HOW TO USE THIS BOOK

To begin, turn to today's calendar date, and fill in the year at the top of the page's first entry. Here, you can record the meaningful minutiae of the day, be it a single nourishing thought, a mindful observation, or an unexpected inspiration—whatever illuminates your own personal path to positive change. On the next day, turn the page and fill in the date accordingly. Do likewise throughout the year. When the year has ended, start the next year in the second entry space on the page, and so on through the remaining years.

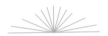

LIVING WELL means something different to each of us, but self-reflection is a valuable tool we all can use to build a healthier life. Whether you measure your wellness in fitness goals or spiritual nourishment, illness management or simple kindness to others, reflecting on your thoughts and actions—and committing to that practice of self-reflection—can bring about powerful positive change. Use this book as a tool for personal growth. Fill it with the encouraging odds and ends of each day, and as the months and years go by, reread your reflections from the past. Witness the blossoming of your best self, and discover what it truly means—to *you*—to live well.

Here are some ways to get started:

- **Reflect on the joys of new beginnings.** Acknowledge the opportunities—in this very moment—for a fresh start.

- **Take note of your self-care rituals.** How many hours did you sleep last night? How many glasses of water did you drink today? How much time did you spend outdoors?

- **Create a new goal, or check in on your past intentions.** Note your successes and progress. Where do you need to renew your commitment?

- **Identify what you learned today.** Consider the encounters and happenings that shape us every day, at every age.

- **Reflect on today's conversations.** What was the inspirational takeaway? Did you overhear something that lifted your spirits? Record a quote, comment or affirmation that gives you hope.

- **Gently acknowledge your struggles.** If you're in pain, what brought you comfort today? How have you grown stronger? How will tomorrow be different?

- **Consider your need for control.** What can you let go of today?

- **Think of those who came before you**—family members, ancestors, and cultures. Who are they, and what can they teach you?

- **Get to know yourself.** What excites you? Where and when are you most content? Notice the moments that bring you peace.

- **Celebrate your relationships.** Who loves you unconditionally? Whom do you trust? With whom would you like to have a conversation right now?

- **Embrace change.** Identify the ways your life is subject to the unknown. What expectations are tying you down? What are you so afraid of?

- **Describe today's "me time."** How did you relax? What did you do to treat yourself? How will you reward yourself tomorrow?

- **Get creative.** Make a bold statement. Explore new forms of self-expression. Define, and redefine, your art of living well.

JANUARY 1

20

20

20

20

20

JANURY 2

20 ·

20

20

20

20

JANUARY 3

2017 | Brooke is still the
cutest.

20

20

20

20

JANURY 4

20

20

20

20

20

JANUARY 5

2017 Today is Ginger's birthday.
Lou got some birthday
cake in honor of her.

20

20

20

20

JANUARY 6

20

20

20

20

20

JANUARY 7

20

20

20

20

20

20

20

20

20

20

JANUARY 9

20

20

20

20

20

JANUARY 10

20

20

20

20

20

20

20

20

20

20

JANUARY 12

20

20

20

20

20

JANUARY 13

20

20

20

20

20

JANUARY 14

20

20

20

20

20

JANURY 15

20

20

20

20

20

JANUARY 16

20

20

20

20

20

JANURY 17

20

20

20

20

20

JANURY 18

20

20

20

20

20

JANUARY 19

20

20

20

20

20

JANUARY 20

20

20

20

20

20

JANUARY 21

20

20

20

20

20

JANURY 22

20

20

20

20

20

JANUARY 23

20

20

20

20

20

JANURARY 24

20

20

20

20

20

JANUARY 25

20

20

20

20

20

JANUARY 26

20

20

20

20

20

JANUARY 27

20

20

20

20

20

JANUARY 28

20

20

20

20

20

JANUARY 29

20

20

20

20

20

JANUARY 30

20

20

20

20

20

JANURARY 31

20

20

20

20

20

FEBRUARY 1

20

20

20

20

20

FEBRUARY 2

20

20

20

20

20

FEBRUARY 3

20

20

20

20

20

FEBRUARY 4

20

20

20

20

20

FEBRUARY 5

20

20

20

20

20

FEBRUARY 6

20

20

20

20

20

FEBRUARY 7

20

20

20

20

20

FEBRUARY 8

20

20

20

20

20

FEBRUARY 9

20

20

20

20

20

FEBRUARY 10

20

20

20

20

20

FEBRUARY 11

20

20

20

20

20

FEBRUARY 12

20

20

20

20

20

FEBRUARY 13

20

20

20

20

20

FEBRUARY 14

20

20

20

20

20

FEBRUARY 15

20

20

20

20

20

FEBRUARY 16

20

20

20

20

20

FEBRUARY 17

....

20

_____

_____

_____

_____

_____

....

20

_____

_____

_____

_____

_____

....

20

_____

_____

_____

_____

_____

....

20

_____

_____

_____

_____

_____

....

20

_____

_____

_____

_____

_____

....

FEBRUARY 18

20

20

20

20

20

FEBRUARY 19

20

20

20

20

20

20

20

20

20

20

20

20

20

20

20

20

20

20

20

20

FEBRUARY 23

20

20

20

20

20

FEBRUARY 24

20

20

20

20

20

FEBRUARY 25

20

20

20

20

20

FEBRUARY 26

20

20

20

20

20

FEBRUARY 27

20

20

20

20

20

FEBRUARY 28

20

20

20

20

20

FEBRUARY 29

20

20

20

20

20

MARCH 1

....

20

_____
_____
_____
_____

....

20

_____
_____
_____
_____

....

20

_____
_____
_____
_____

....

20

_____
_____
_____
_____

....

20

_____
_____
_____
_____

....

MARCH 2

20

20

20

20

20

MARCH 3

20

20

20

20

20

MARCH 4

20

20

20

20

20

MARCH 5

20

20

20

20

20

MARCH 6

20

20

20

20

20

MARCH 7

20

20

20

20

20

20

20

20

20

20

MARCH 9

20

20

20

20

20

MARCH 10

20

20

20

20

20

MARCH 11

20

20

20

20

20

MARCH 12

20

20

20

20

20

MARCH 13

20

20

20

20

20

MARCH 14

20

20

20

20

20

MARCH 15

20

20

20

20

20

MARCH 16

20

20

20

20

20

MARCH 17

20

20

20

20

20

MARCH 18

20

20

20

20

20

MARCH 19

20

20

20

20

20

20

20

20

20

20

MARCH 21

20

20

20

20

20

MARCH 22

20

20

20

20

20

20

20

20

20

20

MARCH 24

20

20

20

20

20

MARCH 25

20

20

20

20

20

20

20

20

20

20

MARCH 27

20

20

20

20

20

MARCH 28

20

20

20

20

20

MARCH 29

20

20

20

20

20

MARCH 30

20

20

20

20

20

MARCH 31

20

20

20

20

20

APRIL 1

20

20

20

20

20

APRIL 2

20

20

20

20

20

APRIL 3

20

20

20

20

20

APRIL 4

20

20

20

20

20

APRIL 5

20

20

20

20

20

APRIL 6

20

20

20

20

20

APRIL 7

20

20

20

20

20

APRIL 8

20

20

20

20

20

20

20

20

20

20

APRIL 10

20

20

20

20

20

APRIL 11

20

20

20

20

20

APRIL 12

20

20

20

20

20

APReIL 13

20

20

20

20

20

20

20

20

20

20

APRIL 15

20

20

20

20

20

APRIL 16

20

20

20

20

20

APRIL 17

20

20

20

20

20

APRIL 18

20

20

20

20

20

20

20

20

20

20

20

20

20

20

20

APRIL 21

20

20

20

20

20

APRIL 22

20

20

20

20

20

20

20

20

20

20

APRIL 24

20

20

20

20

20

APRIL 25

20

20

20

20

20

APRIL 26

20

20

20

20

20

APRIL 27

20

20

20

20

20

APRIL 28

20

20

20

20

20

20

20

20

20

20

APRIL 30

20

20

20

20

20

MAY 1

20

20

20

20

20

MAY 2

20

20

20

20

20

20

20

20

20

20

20

20

20

20

20

MAY 5

20

20

20

20

20

MAY 6

20

20

20

20

20

MAY 7

20

20

20

20

20

20

20

20

20

20

MAY 9

20

20

20

20

20

MAY 10

20

20

20

20

20

MAY 11

20

20

20

20

20

MAY 12

20

20

20

20

20

MAY 13

20

20

20

20

20

MAY 14

20

20

20

20

20

MAY 15

20

20

20

20

20

20

20

20

20

20

20

20

20

20

20

MAY 18

20

20

20

20

20

MAY 19

20

20

20

20

20

20

20

20

20

20

MAY 21

20

20

20

20

20

20

20

20

20

20

20

20

20

20

20

MAY 24

20

20

20

20

20

20

20

20

20

20

MAY 26

20

20

20

20

20

MAY 27

20

20

20

20

20

20

20

20

20

20

MAY 29

20

20

20

20

20

MAY 30

20

20

20

20

20

20

20

20

20

20

JUNE 1

20

20

20

20

20

JUNE 2

20

20

20

20

20

JUNE 3

20

20

20

20

20

JUNE 4

20

20

20

20

20

JUNE 5

20

20

20

20

20

JUNE 6

20

20

20

20

20

20

20

20

20

20

JUNE 8

20

20

20

20

20

JUNE 9

20

20

20

20

20

JUNE 10

20

20

20

20

20

JUNE 11

20

20

20

20

20

JUNE 12

20

20

20

20

20

JUNE 13

20

20

20

20

20

20

20

20

20

20

JUNE 15

20

20

20

20

20

JUNE 16

20

20

20

20

20

JUNE 17

20

20

20

20

20

JUNE 18

20

20

20

20

20

JUNE 19

20

20

20

20

20

JUNE 20

20

20

20

20

20

JUNE 21

20

20

20

20

20

JUNE 22

20

20

20

20

20

JUNE 23

20

20

20

20

20

JUNE 24

20

20

20

20

20

JUNE 25

20

20

20

20

20

JUNE 26

20

20

20

20

20

20

20

20

20

20

JUNE 28

20

20

20

20

20

JUNE 29

20

20

20

20

20

JUNE 30

20

20

20°

20

20

JULY 1

20

20

20

20

20

JULY 2

20

20

20

20

20

JULY 3

20

20

20

20

20

JULY 4

20

20

20

20

20

JULY 5

20

20

20

20

20

JULY 6

20

20

20

20

20

JULY 7

20

20

20

20

20

JULY 8

20

20

20

20

20

JULY 9

20

20

20

20

20

JULY 10

20

20

20

20

20

JULY 11

20

20

20

20

20

20

20

20

20

20

JULY 13

20

20

20

20

20

JULY 14

20

20

20

20

20

JULY 15

20

20

20

20

20

JULY 16

20

20

20

20

20

JULY 17

20

20

20

20

20

JULY 18

20

20

20

20

20

JULY 19

20

20

20

20

20

20

20

20

20

20

JULY 21

20

20

20

20

20

JULY 22

20

20

20

20

20

20

20

20

20

20

JULY 24

2016 Today Aidan & Brooke are Mr & Mrs Congrats from Becca & Matt

20

20

20

20

JULY 25

20

20

20

20

20

JULY 26

20

20

20

20

20

JULY 27

20

20

20

20

20

JULY 28

20

20

20

20

20

JULY 29

20

20

20

20

20

20

20

20

20

20

JULY 31

20

20

20

20

20

AUGUST 1

20

20

20

20

20

AUGUST 2

20

20

20

20

20

AUGUST 3

20

20

20

20

20

AUGUST 4

20

20

20

20

20

AUGUST 5

20

20

20

20

20

AUGUST 6

20

20

20

20

20

AUGUST 7

20

20

20

20

20

AUGUST 8

20

20

20

20

20

AUGUST 9

20

20

20

20

20

AUGUST 10

20

20

20

20

20

AUGUST 11

....

20	

....

20	

....

20	

....

20	

....

20	

....

AUGUST 12

20

20

20

20

20

AUGUST 13

20

20

20

20

20

AUGUST 14

20

20

20

20

20

AUGUST 15

20

20

20

20

20

AUGUST 16

20

20

20

20

20

AUGUST 17

20

20

20

20

20

AUGUST 18

20

20

20

20

20

20

20

20

20

20

AUGUST 20

20

20

20

20

20

AUGUST 21

20

20

20

20

20

AUGUST 22

20

20

20

20

20

AUGUST 23

20

20

20

20

20

AUGUST 24

20

20

20

20

20

AUGUST 25

20

20

20

20

20

AUGUST 26

20

20

20

20

20

AUGUST 27

20

20

20

20

20

AUGUST 28

20

20

20

20

20

AUGUST 29

20

20

20

20

20

AUGUST 30

20

20

20

20

20

AUGUST 31

20

20

20

20

20

SEPTEMBER 1

20

20

20

20

20

SEPTEMBER 2

20

20

20

20

20

SEPTEMBER 3

20

20

20

20

20

20

20

20

20

20

SEPTEMBER 5

20

20

20

20

20

SEPTEMBER 6

20

20

20

20

20

SEPTEMBER 7

20

20

20

20

20

SEPTEMBER 8

20

20

20

20

20

SEPTEMBER 9

20

20

20

20

20

SEPTEMBER 10

20

20

20

20

20

SEPTEMBER 11

20

20

20

20

20

SEPTEMBER 12

20

20

20

20

20

SEPTEMBER 13

20

20

20

20

20

SEPTEMBER 14

20

20

20

20

20

SEPTEMBER 15

20

20

20

20

20

SEPTEMBER 16

20

20

20

20

20

SEPTEMBER 17

20

20

20

20

20

20

20

20

20

20

SEPTEMBER 19

20

20

20

20

20

SEPTEMBER 20

20

20

20

20

20

SEPTEMBER 21

20

20

20

20

20

SEPTEMBER 22

20

20

20

20

20

SEPTEMBER 23

20

20

20

20

20

SEPTEMBER 24

20

20

20

20

20

SEPTEMBER 25

20

20

20

20

20

SEPTEMBER 26

20

20

20

20

20

SEPTEMBER 27

20

20

20

20

20

SEPTEMBER 28

20

20

20

20

20

SEPTEMBER 29

20

20

20

20

20

SEPTEMBER 30

20

20

20

20

20

OCTOBER 1

20

20

20

20

20

OCTOBER 2

20

20

20

20

20

OCTOBER 3

20

20

20

20

20

OCTOBER 4

20

20

20

20

20

OCTOBER 5

20

20

20

20

20

OCTOBER 6

20

20

20

20

20

OCTOBER 7

20

20

20

20

20

OCTOBER 8

20

20

20

20

20

OCTOBER 9

20

20

20

20

20

OCTOBER 10

20

20

20

20

20

OCTOBER 11

20

20

20

20

20

OCTOBER 12

20

20

20

20

20

OCTOBER 13

20

20

20

20

20

OCTOBER 14

20

20

20

20

20

OCTOBER 15

20

20

20

20

20

OCTOBER 16

20

20

20

20

20

OCTOBER 17

20

20

20

20

20

OCTOBER 18

20

20

20

20

20

OCTOBER 19

20

20

20

20

20

OCTOBER 20

20

20

20

20

20

OCTOBER 21

20

20

20

20

20

OCTOBER 22

20

20

20

20

20

OCTOBER 23

20

20

20

20

20

OCTOBER 24

20

20

20

20

20

OCTOBER 25

20

20

20

20

20

OCTOBER 26

20

20

20

20

20

OCTOBER 27

20

20

20

20

20

OCTOBER 28

20

20

20

20

20

OCTOBER 29

20

20

20

20

20

OCTOBER 30

20

20

20

20

20

OCTOBER 31

20

20

20

20

20

NOVEMBER 1

20

20

20

20

20

NOVEMBER 2

20

20

20

20

20

NOVEMBER 3

20

20

20

20

20

NOVEMBER 4

20

20

20

20

20

NOVEMBER 5

20

20

20

20

20

NOVEMBER 6

20

20

20

20

20

NOVEMBER 7

20

20

20

20

20

NOVEMBER 8

20

20

20

20

20

NOVEMBER 9

20

20

20

20

20

NOVEMBER 10

20

20

20

20

20

NOVEMBER 11

20

20

20

20

20

NOVEMBER 12

20

20

20

20

20

NOVEMBER 13

....

20

....

20

....

20

....

20

....

20

....

NOVEMBER 14

20

20

20

20

20

NOVEMBER 15

20

20

20

20

20

NOVEMBER 16

20

20

20

20

20

NOVEMBER 17

20

20

20

20

20

NOVEMBER 18

20

20

20

20

20

NOVEMBER 19

20

20

20

20

20

NOVEMBER 20

20

20

20

20

20

NOVEMBER 21

20

20

20

20

20

NOVEMBER 22

20

20

20

20

20

NOVEMBER 23

20

20

20

20

20

NOVEMBER 24

20

20

20

20

20

NOVEMBER 25

20

20

20

20

20

NOVEMBER 26

20

20

20

20

20

20

20

20

20

20

NOVEMBER 28

20

20

20

20

20

NOVEMBER 29

20

20

20

20

20

NOVEMBER 30

20

20

20

20

20

DECEMBER 1

20

20

20

20

20

DECEMBER 2

20

20

20

20

20

DECEMBER 3

20

20

20

20

20

DECEMBER 4

20

20

20

20

20

DECEMBER 5

20

20

20

20

20

DECEMBER 6

20

20

20

20

20

DECEMBER 7

20

20

20

20

20

DECEMBER 8

20

20

20

20

20

DECEMBER 9

20

20

20

20

20

DECEMBER 10

20

20

20

20

20

DECEMBER 11

20

20

20

20

20

DECEMBER 12

20

20

20

20

20

DECEMBER 13

20

20

20

20

20

DECEMBER 14

20

20

20

20

20

DECEMBER 15

20

20

20

20

20

DECEMBER 16

20

20

20

20

20

DECEMBER 17

20

20

20

20

20

DECEMBER 18

20

20

20

20

20

DECEMBER 19

20

20

20

20

20

DECEMBER 20

20

20

20

20

20

DECEMBER 21

20

20

20

20

20

DECEMBER 22

20

20

20

20

20

DECEMBER 23

20

20

20

20

20

DECEMBER 24

20

20

20

20

20

DECEMBER 25

20

20

20

20

20

DECEMBER 26

20

20

20

20

20

DECEMBER 27

20

20

20

20

20

DECEMBER 28

20

20

20

20

20

DECEMBER 29

20

20

20

20

20

DECEMBER 30

20

20

20

20

20

DECEMBER 31

20

20

20

20

20

DATES TO REMEMBER

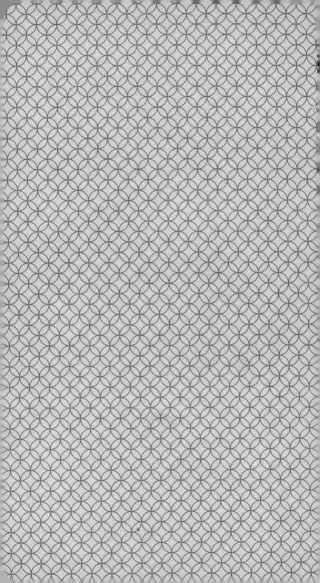